The Ultimate Guide to Nutrition Food for Kids:

A Parent's Handbook

TABLE OF CONTAINS

Chapter 1: Understanding Nutrition for Kids

The Importance of Nutrition for Children

Nutrition is crucial for the growth and development of children, making it essential for parents to prioritize healthy eating habits from a young age. The food choices we make for our children can have a significant impact on their overall health and well-being. By providing them with nutritious meals and snacks, we can help them thrive and reach their full potential.

Organic nutrition food for kids is a great option for parents who want to ensure that their children are consuming food that is free from harmful pesticides and chemicals. Choosing organic fruits, vegetables, and grains can provide children with essential vitamins and minerals while reducing their exposure to potentially harmful substances. By opting for organic options, parents can support their children's health and well-being in a natural and sustainable way.

Vegan nutrition food for kids is another excellent choice for parents looking to provide their children with a plant-based diet rich in nutrients. Vegan foods such as fruits, vegetables, legumes, and whole grains can be a great source of vitamins, minerals, and fiber. By introducing children to a variety of vegan options, parents can help them develop healthy eating habits that can last a lifetime.

Gluten-free nutrition food for kids is essential for children who have gluten sensitivities or allergies. By choosing gluten-free grains such as rice, quinoa, and oats, parents can provide their children with nutritious options that are safe and easy to digest. Gluten-free nutrition food can help children avoid discomfort and potential health issues related to gluten consumption.

Allergy-friendly nutrition food for kids is vital for children with food allergies or sensitivities. By carefully selecting foods that are free from common allergens such as nuts, dairy, and soy, parents can ensure that their children are safe and well-nourished. Allergy-friendly nutrition food can help children thrive and enjoy a variety of delicious and nutritious meals without worrying about potential allergic reactions.

Common Nutritional Needs for Kids

To ensure that your child is healthy and thriving, it is important to understand their common nutritional needs. Kids have unique dietary requirements that must be met for them to grow and develop properly. By providing your child with the right balance of nutrients, you can set them up for a lifetime of good health and wellness.

One of the most important nutritional needs for kids is a diet rich in fruits and vegetables. These foods are packed with essential vitamins, minerals, and antioxidants that support overall health and immunity. Encourage your child to eat a variety of colorful fruits and vegetables each day to ensure they are getting all the nutrients they need. You can also get creative with how you serve these foods to make them more appealing to your child.

Another key nutritional need for kids is protein. Protein is essential for growth, development, and muscle repair. Make sure your child is getting enough protein by including sources such as lean meats, poultry, fish, eggs, dairy products, nuts, and seeds in their diet. You can also incorporate plant-based sources of protein like beans, lentils, tofu, and quinoa to keep things interesting.

Whole grains are also an important component of a child's diet. Whole grains provide fiber, which is important for digestive health, as well as essential vitamins and minerals. Encourage your child to eat a variety of whole grains such as brown rice, quinoa, oats, and whole wheat bread to ensure they are getting all the nutrients they need. You can also incorporate whole grains into snacks and meals to boost their nutritional value.

In addition to these essential nutrients, it is important to focus on hydration. Water is essential for overall health and plays a crucial role in digestion, circulation, and temperature regulation. Encourage your child to drink plenty of water throughout the day to stay hydrated and healthy. You can also offer water-rich foods like fruits and vegetables to help meet their hydration needs. By focusing on these common nutritional needs for kids, you can help your child grow and thrive in a healthy and sustainable way.

How Nutrition Affects Growth and Development

Nutrition plays a crucial role in the growth and development of children. The food that kids consume daily not only fuels their bodies but also provides essential nutrients that are needed for proper growth and development. By focusing on providing nutritious and balanced meals, parents can help support their children's overall health and well-being.

One of the keyways that nutrition affects growth and development is through the intake of essential vitamins and minerals. Nutrients such as calcium, vitamin D, and iron are vital for bone health, immune function, and overall growth. By incorporating a variety of fruits, vegetables, whole grains, and lean proteins into their diets, parents can ensure that their children are getting the nutrients they need to thrive.

In addition to vitamins and minerals, the types of foods that children eat can also impact their development. For example, foods high in sugar and unhealthy fats can lead to weight gain and other health issues, while foods that are rich in antioxidants and fiber can help support brain function and digestion. By choosing nutrient-dense foods that are low in added sugars and unhealthy fats, parents can help set their children up for success.

It's also important to consider any food allergies or sensitivities that children may have when planning meals. By choosing allergy-friendly options and avoiding common allergens, parents can help prevent adverse reactions and support their children's overall health. Additionally, incorporating probiotic-rich foods into their diets can help support a healthy gut microbiome and boost immune function.

Overall, by focusing on providing nutritious, balanced meals that are free from harmful additives and allergens, parents can help support their children's growth and development. By making informed choices about the foods, they serve and prioritizing their children's health, parents can set their kids up for a lifetime of good eating habits and overall wellness. Remember, every bite counts when it comes to nourishing your child's body and mind.

Chapter 2: Organic Nutrition Food for Kids

Benefits of Organic Foods for Children

Organic foods are a great choice for children due to their numerous benefits. From fruits and vegetables to dairy products and grains, organic foods are grown without the use of synthetic pesticides, hormones, or antibiotics. This means that your child is getting food that is free from harmful chemicals and additives, making it a healthier option overall.

One of the key benefits of organic foods for children is their higher nutritional value. Studies have shown that organic fruits and vegetables contain higher levels of vitamins, minerals, and antioxidants compared to conventionally grown produce. This means that your child is getting more nutrients with each bite, helping to support their overall health and development.

In addition to being more nutritious, organic foods are also better for the environment. Organic farming practices focus on sustainability and reducing the impact on the planet, making them an eco-friendlier choice. By choosing organic foods for your child, you are not only supporting their health but also helping to protect the environment for future generations.

Furthermore, organic foods are often fresher and tastier than their non-organic counterparts. This is because they are grown in nutrient-rich soil and harvested at the peak of ripeness, resulting in better flavor and texture. By introducing your child to organic foods, you are helping them develop a palate for fresh, wholesome ingredients that will set them up for a lifetime of healthy eating habits.

Overall, the benefits of organic foods for children are vast and undeniable. From improved nutrition and environmental sustainability to better taste and freshness, organic foods are a great choice for parents looking to provide their child with the best possible start in life. So why not make the switch to organic today and give your child the gift of health and wellness?

How to Identify Organic Products

Organic products are becoming more popular these days, but how do you know if a product is truly organic? It's important to be able to identify organic products so that you can make the best choices for your family's health. Here are some tips on how to identify organic products:

1. Look for the USDA Organic seal: One of the easiest ways to identify organic products is to look for the USDA Organic seal. This seal indicates that the product has been certified as organic by the United States Department of Agriculture. Products with this seal have met strict guidelines for organic production, including the use of organic ingredients and no synthetic pesticides or fertilizers.

2. Read the ingredients list: Another way to identify organic products is to read the ingredients list. Organic products will typically have a short list of ingredients that are easy to pronounce and recognize. Look for ingredients like organic fruits, vegetables, grains, and meats. Avoid products with long lists of artificial ingredients or preservatives.

3. Check for third-party certifications: In addition to the USDA Organic seal, there are other third-party certifications that can help you identify organic products.

Look for certifications like Non-GMO Project Verified, Certified Organic by Oregon Tilth, or Certified Humane. These certifications indicate that the product has been verified as organic by an independent organization.

4. Look for local and small-scale producers: Another way to identify organic products is to buy from local and small-scale producers. These producers are more likely to use organic practices and prioritize the health of their customers and the environment. Look for products at farmers markets, co-ops, or directly from the producer.

5. Be wary of greenwashing: Finally, be wary of greenwashing – marketing tactics that make a product appear more organic or environmentally friendly than it actually is. Look for specific certifications and do your own research to ensure that a product is truly organic. By following these tips, you can easily identify organic products and make the best choices for your family's health.

Organic Meal Planning for Kids

Organic meal planning for kids is a great way to ensure that your little ones are getting the best nutrition possible. By choosing organic ingredients, you are avoiding harmful pesticides and chemicals that can be found in conventionally grown produce. This can help to keep your children healthy and thriving, both now and in the future.

When planning organic meals for kids, it's important to focus on a variety of fruits, vegetables, whole grains, and lean proteins. By incorporating a rainbow of colors into their meals, you can ensure that they are getting a wide range of vitamins and minerals. Try to include different textures and flavors to keep things interesting and appealing to your children's taste buds.

One great way to get your kids involved in organic meal planning is to take them to the farmer's market or grocery store with you. Let them pick out fruits and vegetables that catch their eye and involve them in the cooking process. When children feel like they have a say in what they are eating, they are more likely to try new foods and develop healthy eating habits.

In addition to focusing on organic ingredients, it's also important to consider other factors such as food allergies and sensitivities. If your child has gluten intolerance or a dairy allergy, there are plenty of organic and allergy-friendly options available. By being mindful of your child's specific needs, you can create delicious and nutritious meals that work for your family.

Remember, organic meal planning for kids doesn't have to be complicated or time-consuming. With a little creativity and planning, you can provide your children with nourishing and delicious meals that will support their growth and development. By making healthy eating a priority in your household, you are setting your children up for a lifetime of good health.

Chapter 3: Vegan Nutrition Food for Kids

Plant-Based Sources of Essential Nutrients

Plant-based sources of essential nutrients are a fantastic way to ensure your child is getting all the vitamins and minerals they need to thrive. Whether your child follows a vegan diet or simply enjoys incorporating more plant-based options into their meals, there are plenty of delicious and nutritious options to choose from.

One of the most important nutrients for growing children is calcium, which is essential for building strong bones and teeth. Luckily, there are plenty of plant-based sources of calcium, such as broccoli, kale, almonds, and fortified plant-based milks. These foods are not only delicious but also packed with the nutrients your child needs to grow up healthy and strong.

Iron is another essential nutrient that can be found in plant-based foods. Foods such as lentils, chickpeas, tofu, and quinoa are all excellent sources of iron, which is important for healthy blood cells and overall growth and development. By incorporating these foods into your child's diet, you can ensure they are getting all the iron they need to thrive.

Omega-3 fatty acids are crucial for brain development and function and can be found in plant-based sources such as flaxseeds, chia seeds, walnuts, and hemp seeds. These foods are not only packed with omega-3s, but also provide a healthy dose of fiber and protein to keep your child feeling full and satisfied.

Incorporating plant-based sources of essential nutrients into your child's diet is a great way to ensure they are getting all the vitamins and minerals they need to grow up healthy and strong. By including foods such as calcium-rich broccoli, iron-packed lentils, and omega-3-rich chia seeds, you can help your child thrive on a plant-based diet. So get creative in the kitchen and experiment with new and exciting plant-based foods to keep your child happy, healthy, and nourished.

Creating Balanced Vegan Meals for Children

Creating balanced vegan meals for children is not as daunting as it may seem. With a little bit of planning and creativity, you can ensure that your child is getting all the nutrients they need to thrive on a plant-based diet. One key to success is to include a variety of foods from all the food groups to ensure a well-rounded diet. This means incorporating fruits, vegetables, whole grains, legumes, nuts, and seeds into your child's meals.

When planning meals for your child, it's important to consider their specific nutritional needs. Children need a variety of nutrients to support their growth and development, including protein, iron, calcium, vitamin D, and vitamin B12. Luckily, all these nutrients can be found in plant-based foods. To ensure that your child is getting enough of these nutrients, include a variety of protein sources such as beans, lentils, tofu, tempeh, and quinoa, as well as fortified plant-based milks and cereals.

In addition to including a variety of foods from all the food groups, it's also important to pay attention to portion sizes. Children have smaller stomachs than adults, so it's important to offer them smaller, more frequent meals and snacks throughout the day. This will help to ensure that they are getting enough calories and nutrients to support their growth and development.

Another tip for creating balanced vegan meals for children is to get them involved in the meal planning and preparation process. This can help to get them excited about trying new foods and flavors and can also help them to develop a positive relationship with food. Encourage your child to help choose recipes, shop for ingredients, and even help in the kitchen.

Overall, creating balanced vegan meals for children is all about balance, variety, and creativity. By including a variety of foods from all the food groups, paying attention to portion sizes, and getting your child involved in the process, you can ensure that they are getting all the nutrients they need to thrive on a plant-based diet. Remember, every meal is an opportunity to nourish your child's body and mind, so have fun with it and enjoy the process!

Vegan Snack Ideas for Kids

Are you looking for healthy and delicious snack ideas for your kids that are vegan-friendly? Look no further! In this subchapter, we will explore some creative and nutritious vegan snack options that your kids will love. These snacks are not only tasty but also packed with essential nutrients to support your child's growth and development.

One simple and nutritious vegan snack idea for kids is to make fruit kabobs. Simply skewer a variety of colorful fruits such as strawberries, blueberries, pineapple, and grapes onto wooden skewers. These fruit kabobs are not only visually appealing but also a fun and easy way to get your kids to eat more fruit. You can also serve them with a side of dairy-free yogurt for dipping.

Another great vegan snack idea for kids is homemade trail mix. Mix a variety of nuts, seeds, dried fruits, and even some dairy-free chocolate chips for a delicious and satisfying snack. You can customize the trail mix to your child's preferences and even add in some superfoods like chia seeds or goji berries for an extra nutritional boost.

For a savory vegan snack option, consider making homemade hummus with veggie sticks. Hummus is a creamy and flavorful dip made from chickpeas, tahini, lemon juice, and garlic. Serve it with a variety of fresh vegetable sticks such as carrots, cucumbers, bell peppers, and cherry tomatoes for a crunchy and satisfying snack. This snack is not only delicious but also packed with protein, fiber, and vitamins.

If your kids have a sweet tooth, try making vegan banana oat cookies. These cookies are made from ripe bananas, rolled oats, and a touch of sweetness from maple syrup or dates. They are easy to make and can be customized with add-ins like chocolate chips, nuts, or dried fruits. These cookies are a healthier alternative to traditional store-bought cookies and are perfect for satisfying your child's sweet cravings.

In conclusion, there are plenty of delicious and nutritious vegan snack options for kids that are easy to prepare and will keep your little ones satisfied and energized throughout the day. By incorporating these snacks into your child's diet, you can help them develop healthy eating habits and support their overall well-being. So why not get creative in the kitchen and whip up some of these tasty vegan snacks for your kids today?

Chapter 4: Gluten-Free Nutrition Food for Kids

Understanding Gluten Sensitivities in Children

Understanding gluten sensitivities in children is crucial for parents who want to ensure their little ones are happy and healthy. Gluten is a protein found in wheat, barley, and rye that can cause adverse reactions in some children. It's important to be aware of the symptoms of gluten sensitivity, which can include stomach pain, bloating, diarrhea, and fatigue. By being informed and proactive, parents can help their children avoid discomfort and potential long-term health issues associated with gluten sensitivities.

For children with gluten sensitivities, it's essential to find alternative food options that are safe and nutritious. Luckily, there are many gluten-free products available on the market today, making it easier than ever to accommodate your child's dietary needs. From gluten-free bread and pasta to snacks and desserts, there are plenty of delicious options to choose from. By incorporating these gluten-free alternatives into your child's diet, you can ensure they are still getting the nutrients they need without compromising their health.

In addition to avoiding gluten-containing foods, it's also important to focus on incorporating nutrient-dense, whole foods into your child's diet. This includes fruits, vegetables, lean proteins, and healthy fats. These foods not only provide essential vitamins and minerals but also support overall health and well-being. By prioritizing whole foods, you can help boost your child's immune system, improve their digestion, and support their brain development.

When it comes to gluten sensitivities in children, it's important to remember that every child is unique. Some children may have severe reactions to gluten, while others may only experience mild symptoms. It's crucial to work with a healthcare provider to determine the best course of action for your child. This may involve undergoing testing to confirm gluten sensitivity or working with a nutritionist to create a personalized meal plan that meets your child's specific needs.

Overall, understanding gluten sensitivities in children is an important step in promoting their overall health and well-being. By being proactive, informed, and supportive, parents can help their children thrive despite dietary restrictions. With the right knowledge and resources, you can ensure that your child has access to delicious, nutritious foods that support their growth and development. Remember, you're not alone in this journey – there are plenty of resources and support available to help you navigate gluten sensitivities in children with confidence and positivity.

Gluten-Free Substitutes for Kids' Favorite Foods

Are you looking for gluten-free substitutes for your kids' favorite foods? Look no further! In this subchapter, we will explore some delicious and nutritious alternatives that will keep your little ones happy and healthy. Whether your child has a gluten intolerance, or you simply want to incorporate more gluten-free options into their diet, these suggestions are sure to please even the pickiest of eaters.

One popular gluten-free substitute for kids' favorite foods is almond flour. This versatile ingredient can be used in place of traditional wheat flour in a variety of recipes, from pancakes and muffins to cookies and cakes. Almond flour is not only gluten-free, but it is also rich in protein and fiber, making it a nutritious choice for growing bodies. Your kids won't even notice the difference in taste!

Another great gluten-free substitute is quinoa. This ancient grain is packed with protein, fiber, and essential vitamins and minerals, making it a superfood for kids. Quinoa can be used in place of rice or pasta in dishes like stir-fries, salads, and casseroles. Your kids will love the nutty flavor and fluffy texture of quinoa, and you can feel good knowing they are getting a healthy dose of nutrients with each bite.

For a sweet treat that is gluten-free, try using coconut flour in your baking. Coconut flour is made from dried coconut meat and is a great alternative to traditional wheat flour. It is high in fiber and low in carbohydrates, making it a healthier option for kids with gluten sensitivities. Use coconut flour to make gluten-free cookies, cupcakes, and muffins that your kids will love.

If your kids love pasta but can't have gluten, consider trying spiralized vegetables as a gluten-free alternative. Zucchini, sweet potatoes, and carrots can all be spiralized into noodle-like shapes that make a fun and nutritious base for pasta dishes. Top your veggie noodles with a homemade tomato sauce or pesto for a delicious gluten-free meal that your kids will gobble up.

Incorporating gluten-free substitutes into your kids' favorite foods is easier than you think. With a little creativity and experimentation, you can create delicious and nutritious meals that will keep your kids happy and healthy. So go ahead and give these gluten-free alternatives a try – your kids will thank you for it!

Gluten-Free Meal Prep for Busy Parents

Are you a busy parent struggling to find the time to prepare healthy, gluten-free meals for your kids? Look no further! In this subchapter, we will provide you with some helpful tips and tricks for gluten-free meal prep that will save you time and stress in the kitchen.

First and foremost, it's important to stock your kitchen with gluten-free staples such as quinoa, rice, gluten-free oats, and a variety of gluten-free flours. Having these items on hand will make it easier to whip up quick and nutritious meals for your little ones.

When planning your meals for the week, try to choose recipes that can easily be made in bulk and stored in the fridge or freezer. This will not only save you time during the week, but it will also ensure that you always have a healthy gluten-free option on hand for your kids to enjoy.

Consider investing in some meal prep containers to help you portion out your meals in advance. This will make it easy to grab a pre-made meal from the fridge or freezer when you're short of time or energy. Plus, having meals ready to go will help you resist the temptation to reach for unhealthy convenience foods when you're feeling frazzled.

Remember, meal prep doesn't have to be overwhelming or time-consuming. By taking a little bit of time each week to plan and prepare your meals in advance, you can ensure that your kids are eating nutritious, gluten-free meals that will keep them happy and healthy. So, roll up your sleeves, put on your apron, and get ready to conquer meal prep like a boss!

Chapter 5: Allergy-Friendly Nutrition Food for Kids

Common Food Allergies in Children

Food allergies are becoming increasingly common in children, with some estimates suggesting that up to 8% of children have a food allergy. The most common food allergies in children include milk, eggs, peanuts, tree nuts, soy, wheat, fish, and shellfish. It's important for parents to be aware of these common food allergies and to take steps to ensure that their children are not exposed to these allergens.

One of the best ways to prevent food allergies in children is to introduce a wide variety of foods early on in their diet. By exposing children to a diverse range of foods, you can help to reduce the likelihood of developing allergies later in life. It's also important to be aware of any family history of food allergies, as children with a family history of allergies are more likely to develop allergies themselves.

If you suspect that your child may have a food allergy, it's important to consult with a healthcare professional for a proper diagnosis. Common symptoms of food allergies in children include hives, itching, swelling, difficulty breathing, and digestive issues. If your child experiences any of these symptoms after eating a particular food, it's important to eliminate that food from their diet and seek medical advice.

In addition to avoiding common allergens, there are also a few alternative foods that can help to nourish children with food allergies. For example, almond milk or coconut milk can be used as a substitute for cow's milk, and sunflower seed butter or soy butter can be used as a substitute for peanut butter. It's important to read food labels carefully and to be vigilant about cross-contamination when preparing meals for children with food allergies.

By being proactive and informed about common food allergies in children, parents can help to ensure that their children are healthy and thriving. With the right knowledge and resources, it's possible to provide children with nutritious and delicious meals that cater to their specific dietary needs. Remember, prevention is key when it comes to food allergies, so be sure to stay educated and take the necessary steps to keep your child safe and healthy.

Allergy-Friendly Cooking Tips for Parents

Are you a parent struggling to navigate the world of allergy-friendly cooking for your child? Fear not, for this subchapter provides you with practical tips and advice to make mealtime a breeze. Whether your child has a nut allergy, gluten intolerance, or any other dietary restriction, we've got you covered with delicious and nutritious recipes that are safe for them to enjoy.

One of the most important things to keep in mind when cooking for a child with allergies is to always read labels carefully. Make sure to check for any potential allergens in all ingredients, including spices and condiments. It's also a good idea to double-check labels each time you purchase a product, as ingredients and manufacturing processes can change.

When it comes to meal planning, try to focus on whole, unprocessed foods that are naturally free of allergens. Fruits, vegetables, lean proteins, and whole grains are great options that can be easily tailored to fit your child's dietary needs. Get creative with your cooking by experimenting with different herbs and spices to add flavor without relying on common allergens like dairy or nuts.

Another helpful tip is to batch cook and freeze meals in advance. This can save you time and stress on busy weeknights when you're short of time. Simply defrost and reheat a pre-prepared meal, and you'll have a delicious and allergy-friendly dinner on the table in no time. Additionally, involving your child in the cooking process can help them feel empowered and excited about trying new foods.

Remember, cooking for a child with allergies can be challenging, but with the right tools and resources, you can create delicious and nutritious meals that will keep them healthy and happy. Don't be afraid to get creative in the kitchen and experiment with new ingredients and recipes. Your child will thank you for providing them with safe and satisfying meals that cater to their dietary needs.

Nutritious Alternatives for Allergy-Prone Kids

Are you a parent of a child who suffers from allergies and struggles to find nutritious alternatives for their diet? Look no further! In this subchapter, we will explore some fantastic options for allergy-prone kids that are not only delicious but also packed with essential nutrients to support their growth and development.

One of the best ways to ensure your child is getting the necessary nutrients while avoiding allergens is by opting for organic nutrition food. Organic fruits and vegetables are free from harmful pesticides and chemicals that can trigger allergic reactions in sensitive individuals. By choosing organic options, you can provide your child with wholesome and nutritious meals that support their overall health and well-being.

For parents looking to eliminate animal products from their child's diet, vegan nutrition food is an excellent choice. Plant-based sources of protein, such as beans, lentils, and tofu, can provide essential nutrients without the risk of triggering allergies. Additionally, vegan nutrition food is rich in vitamins, minerals, and antioxidants that support a strong immune system and promote optimal growth and development in children.

If your child has gluten sensitivity or allergy, gluten-free nutrition food is the way to go. Gluten can be found in many common foods, such as bread, pasta, and cereal, but there are plenty of delicious alternatives available that are free from gluten. Look for gluten-free grains like quinoa, rice, and oats to provide your child with energy and essential nutrients without the risk of triggering allergies.

For allergy-friendly options that are packed with nutrients, consider incorporating superfoods into your child's diet. Superfoods like berries, leafy greens, and nuts are rich in antioxidants, vitamins, and minerals that support a healthy immune system and brain function. By including these nutrient-dense foods in your child's meals, you can help them thrive and grow strong.

In conclusion, there are plenty of nutritious alternatives available for allergy-prone kids that can support their overall health and well-being. Whether you choose organic, vegan, gluten-free, superfood, or other allergy-friendly options, it is essential to prioritize your child's nutritional needs and provide them with meals that are both delicious and beneficial. With a little creativity and planning, you can ensure that your child gets the nutrients they need to thrive and live a healthy, happy life.

Chapter 6: Superfood Nutrition Food for Kids

Introducing Superfoods into Kids' Diets

Are you looking to boost your child's health and well-being through nutrition? One great way to do this is by introducing superfoods into their diets. Superfoods are nutrient-dense foods that are packed with vitamins, minerals, antioxidants, and other essential nutrients that can help support your child's overall health. In this subchapter, we will explore the benefits of incorporating superfoods into your child's diet and provide tips on how to make it fun and easy for them to enjoy these nutritious foods.

Superfoods are a great way to ensure that your child is getting the nutrients they need to thrive. From immune-boosting berries like blueberries and strawberries to brain-boosting nuts like almonds and walnuts, there is a wide variety of superfoods that can help support your child's growth and development. By incorporating these nutrient-dense foods into their diet, you can help to provide them with the essential nutrients they need to stay healthy and strong.

One of the best ways to introduce superfoods into your child's diet is by making it fun and exciting for them. Get creative in the kitchen by incorporating superfoods into their favorite dishes or snacks. For example, you can make a delicious smoothie bowl with superfood toppings like chia seeds and goji berries or bake homemade granola bars with nutrient-rich ingredients like oats and flaxseeds. By making superfoods a part of their everyday meals, you can help to instill healthy eating habits that will last a lifetime.

Another great way to introduce superfoods into your child's diet is by getting them involved in the process. Take them grocery shopping with you and let them pick out their favorite superfoods to include in their meals. You can also involve them in meal prep and cooking, allowing them to see firsthand how nutritious and delicious these foods can be. By empowering your child to make healthy food choices, you can help to set them up for a lifetime of good health and well-being.

In conclusion, introducing superfoods into your child's diet is a great way to support their overall health and well-being. By incorporating nutrient-dense foods like berries, nuts, seeds, and leafy greens into their meals, you can help to provide them with the essential nutrients they need to thrive. Make it fun and exciting for them by getting creative in the kitchen and involving them in the process. By instilling healthy eating habits early on, you can help to set your child up for a lifetime of good health and wellness.

Superfood Smoothie Recipes for Picky Eaters

Are you struggling to get your picky eater to consume nutrient-dense foods? Look no further! In this subchapter, we will explore superfood smoothie recipes that are not only delicious but also packed with essential nutrients to support your child's growth and development. These recipes are perfect for kids who are picky eaters, as they can easily disguise the taste of certain vegetables and other healthy ingredients. Let's dive in and discover some exciting new ways to boost your child's nutrition intake!

First up, we have a Green Monster Smoothie that is sure to be a hit with even the pickiest of eaters. This smoothie is packed with leafy greens like spinach and kale, which are rich in vitamins and minerals. To sweeten it up, you can add some banana, pineapple, or mango. The natural sweetness of these fruits will mask the taste of the greens, making it a delicious and nutritious treat for your little one.

Next, try our Berry Blast Smoothie, which is bursting with antioxidants and immune-boosting properties. This smoothie combines a mix of berries such as strawberries, blueberries, and raspberries, along with a splash of almond milk and a dollop of Greek yogurt. Not only is this smoothie delicious, but it also provides a healthy dose of vitamins and minerals to support your child's overall health.

If your child has a sweet tooth, our Chocolate Banana Smoothie is the perfect option. This smoothie combines ripe bananas, cacao powder, almond butter, and a hint of honey for a decadent treat that is still packed with nutrients. The bananas provide a good source of potassium, while the cacao powder offers antioxidants and a rich chocolate flavor that kids will love.

For a refreshing and hydrating option, try our Tropical Paradise Smoothie. This smoothie combines coconut water, pineapple, mango, and a splash of lime juice for a tropical twist that is sure to transport your child to a sunny beach. Not only is this smoothie delicious, but it also provides a good source of electrolytes and hydration, making it a perfect option for active kids.

Incorporating these superfood smoothie recipes into your child's diet is a simple and effective way to boost their nutrition intake and support their overall health. Encourage your picky eater to try new flavors and ingredients by making smoothies together as a fun and interactive activity. With a little creativity and some delicious recipes on hand, you can help your child develop healthy eating habits that will last a lifetime.

Incorporating Superfoods into Everyday Meals

Incorporating superfoods into everyday meals is a great way to boost the nutritional value of your child's diet. Superfoods are nutrient-dense foods that are packed with vitamins, minerals, and antioxidants, making them an excellent addition to any meal. By incorporating superfoods into your child's diet, you can help support their overall health and well-being.

One easy way to incorporate superfoods into everyday meals is by adding them to smoothies. Berries, such as blueberries and strawberries, are excellent superfoods that can be easily blended into a delicious smoothie for your child to enjoy. You can also add leafy greens, such as spinach or kale, to give your child an extra boost of vitamins and minerals.

Another way to incorporate superfoods into everyday meals is by incorporating them into snacks. Nuts and seeds, such as almonds and chia seeds, are great superfoods that can be easily added to homemade granola bars or trail mix for a healthy and satisfying snack. You can also incorporate superfoods into baked goods, such as adding flaxseed or hemp hearts to muffins or cookies.

When planning meals for your child, be sure to include a variety of superfoods to ensure they are getting a wide range of nutrients. Quinoa, sweet potatoes, and avocados are all superfoods that can be easily incorporated into meals such as salads, stir-fries, and wraps. By including a variety of superfoods in your child's diet, you can help support their immune system, brain function, and overall health.

Overall, incorporating superfoods into everyday meals is a simple and effective way to ensure your child is getting the nutrients they need to thrive. By making small changes to your child's diet and incorporating superfoods into their meals, you can help support their overall health and well-being. So why not start incorporating superfoods into your child's meals today and watch them thrive!

Chapter 7: Immune-Boosting Nutrition Food for Kids

Foods that Support a Healthy Immune System

Having a strong immune system is crucial for overall health and well-being, especially for kids. In this subchapter, we will explore some of the best foods that can help support a healthy immune system in children. By incorporating these immune-boosting foods into your child's diet, you can help them stay healthy and ward off illnesses.

One of the best foods for supporting a healthy immune system is fruits and vegetables. These foods are packed with vitamins, minerals, and antioxidants that can help strengthen the immune system. Some of the best immune-boosting fruits and vegetables include oranges, strawberries, blueberries, spinach, and broccoli. Encourage your child to eat a variety of colorful fruits and vegetables every day to ensure they are getting a wide range of nutrients.

In addition to fruits and vegetables, lean proteins such as chicken, turkey, and fish are also important for a healthy immune system. Proteins are essential for building and repairing tissues, including those in the immune system. Make sure your child is getting an adequate amount of protein in their diet to support their immune system.

Another important food for a healthy immune system is yogurt. Yogurt is a great source of probiotics, which are beneficial bacteria that can help support the immune system. Choose plain yogurt with live and active cultures to ensure your child is getting the most benefits. You can also add fruit or honey to sweeten it naturally.

Lastly, incorporating whole grains such as brown rice, quinoa, and oats into your child's diet can also help support a healthy immune system. Whole grains are rich in fiber, vitamins, and minerals that can help boost the immune system. Encourage your child to choose whole grain options over refined grains for maximum immune-boosting benefits. By incorporating these immune-boosting foods into your child's diet, you can help support their overall health and well-being.

Immune-Boosting Recipes for Kids

In this subchapter, we will explore some immune-boosting recipes that are not only delicious but also packed with nutrients to keep your kids healthy and strong. These recipes are perfect for picky eaters and will help support their immune system, especially during cold and flu season.

First up, we have a vibrant and refreshing immune-boosting smoothie. Simply blend some spinach, kale, frozen berries, a banana, and a scoop of immune-boosting superfoods like spirulina or chlorella. This smoothie is not only packed with vitamins and minerals but also tastes great, making it a perfect snack or breakfast option for your little ones.

Next, we have a hearty and comforting immune-boosting soup. Start by sautéing some garlic, onion, and ginger in a pot, then add in some chopped vegetables like carrots, celery, and sweet potatoes. Pour in some vegetable broth and let it simmer until the vegetables are tender. Add in some immune-boosting herbs and spices like turmeric and oregano for an extra kick of flavor and nutrition.

For a fun and interactive immune-boosting snack, try making homemade probiotic-rich yogurt popsicles. Simply blend some plain yogurt, honey, and your child's favorite fruits like strawberries or blueberries. Pour the mixture into popsicle molds and freeze until solid. These popsicles are not only delicious but also packed with good bacteria to support your child's immune system.

If your child has a sweet tooth, try making immune-boosting gummy bears using gelatin, honey, and freshly squeezed orange juice. These gummies are a fun and tasty way to boost your child's immune system while satisfying their cravings for something sweet. You can also add in some chopped fruits for an extra burst of flavor and nutrition.

Incorporating these immune-boosting recipes into your child's diet can help support their overall health and well-being. With a little creativity and a lot of love, you can provide your kids with nutritious and delicious meals that will keep them happy and healthy. So don't be afraid to get creative in the kitchen and have fun experimenting with new flavors and ingredients to create immune-boosting meals that your kids will love.

Tips for Keeping Kids Healthy During Cold and Flu Season

As a parent, it can be challenging to keep your kids healthy during cold and flu season. However, there are some simple tips you can follow to ensure your children stay strong and immune-boosted all year round. By incorporating these strategies into your daily routine, you can help prevent sickness and keep your little ones feeling their best.

First and foremost, it's essential to focus on nutrition food for kids. Make sure your children are getting a balanced diet rich in fruits, vegetables, whole grains, and lean proteins. By providing them with the necessary vitamins and minerals, you can support their immune system and help them fight off any potential illnesses.

Consider incorporating organic nutrition food for kids into their meals whenever possible. Organic foods are free from harmful pesticides and chemicals, making them a healthier option for your children. By choosing organic fruits, vegetables, and meats, you can ensure that your kids are getting the best possible nutrition without any added toxins.

For those with specific dietary needs, such as vegan, gluten-free, or allergy-friendly diets, there are plenty of options available to keep your kids healthy. Look for superfood nutrition food for kids that are packed with nutrients and antioxidants to support their overall health. These foods can help boost their immune system and keep them feeling energized throughout the day.

In addition to focusing on nutrition, consider incorporating probiotic-rich foods into your children's diet. Probiotics are beneficial bacteria that can help support gut health and strengthen the immune system. Foods like yogurt, kefir, and fermented vegetables are excellent sources of probiotics and can help keep your kids healthy during cold and flu season. By following these tips and making healthy choices for your children, you can help them stay strong and resilient in the face of illness. Remember, prevention is key when it comes to keeping your kids healthy, so be proactive and make their well-being a top priority.

Chapter 8: Brain-Boosting Nutrition Food for Kids

Nutrients that Support Cognitive Function in Children

Nutrition plays a crucial role in supporting cognitive function in children. As parents, it is important to ensure that our little ones are getting the nutrients they need to thrive both physically and mentally. In this subchapter, we will discuss the key nutrients that are essential for supporting brain health and cognitive function in children.

First and foremost, omega-3 fatty acids are vital for brain development and function. Foods rich in omega-3s, such as fatty fishlike salmon and mackerel, as well as chia seeds and walnuts, can help support cognitive function in children. Consider incorporating these foods into your child's diet on a regular basis to promote healthy brain development.

In addition to omega-3 fatty acids, antioxidants are also important for cognitive function. Antioxidant-rich foods like berries, dark leafy greens, and dark chocolate can help protect the brain from oxidative stress and improve cognitive function. Encourage your child to eat a variety of colorful fruits and vegetables to ensure they are getting a good mix of antioxidants in their diet.

Furthermore, vitamin E is another nutrient that is essential for brain health. Foods like almonds, sunflower seeds, and spinach are rich sources of vitamin E and can help support cognitive function in children. Including these foods in your child's meals and snacks can help ensure they are getting enough of this important nutrient.

Lastly, it is important to remember the importance of hydration in supporting cognitive function. Dehydration can impair cognitive function, so make sure your child is drinking plenty of water throughout the day. Encourage them to choose water over sugary drinks to keep their brains hydrated and functioning at their best.

Overall, by focusing on incorporating nutrient-dense foods like omega-3 fatty acids, antioxidants, vitamin E, and staying hydrated, you can help support cognitive function in your children. Remember, a healthy diet is key to helping your little ones thrive both physically and mentally.

Brain-Boosting Snacks for School and Playtime

Are you looking for delicious and nutritious snacks to fuel your child's brain during school and playtime? Look no further! In this subchapter, we will explore some brain-boosting snacks that are perfect for kids of all ages. These snacks not only taste great but also provide essential nutrients to support cognitive function and focus.

One of the best brain-boosting snacks for kids is nuts and seeds. These crunchy treats are packed with healthy fats, protein, and antioxidants that support brain health. Almonds, walnuts, and pumpkin seeds are excellent choices for a quick and easy snack that will keep your child energized throughout the day. You can also mix in some dried fruit for a sweet and satisfying treat.

Another great brain-boosting snack option is yogurt with fresh berries. Yogurt is rich in probiotics, which are beneficial for gut health and can have a positive impact on cognitive function. Berries, such as blueberries and strawberries, are loaded with antioxidants that help protect the brain from oxidative stress. This simple snack is not only delicious but also provides a powerful nutritional boost for your child's brain.

For a fun and interactive snack that will keep your child engaged, try making homemade trail mix. Mix a variety of nuts, seeds, dried fruit, and dark chocolate chips for a tasty and nutritious treat. You can customize the trail mix to include your child's favorite ingredients, making it a personalized snack that they will love. This snack is perfect for on-the-go and can be easily packed in a lunchbox or backpack for school or playtime.

If your child has a sweet tooth, consider making homemade energy balls. These bite-sized treats are made with ingredients like oats, nut butter, and honey, and can be customized with add-ins like chia seeds, flaxseeds, or mini chocolate chips. Energy balls are a great source of fiber, protein, and healthy fats, making them a satisfying snack that will keep your child full and focused. Plus, they are easy to make in advance and can be stored in the fridge for quick and convenient snacking.

In conclusion, providing your child with brain-boosting snacks is essential for supporting their cognitive function and overall well-being. By incorporating nuts, seeds, yogurt, berries, trail mix, and energy balls into their diet, you can ensure that they are getting the nutrients they need to thrive. These snacks are not only nutritious but also delicious, making them a hit with kids of all ages. So why not give these brain-boosting snacks a try and watch as your child's focus and energy levels soar!

Meal Ideas to Fuel Growing Minds

Mealtime is not just about filling bellies; it's about fueling growing minds! As parents, we understand the importance of providing our children with nutritious food that will help them thrive both physically and mentally. In this subchapter, we will explore some meal ideas that are not only delicious but also packed with the nutrients needed to support your child's development.

One great option to consider is a hearty breakfast bowl filled with whole grains, fresh fruits, nuts, and seeds. This powerhouse meal will provide your child with a good balance of carbohydrates, protein, and healthy fats to kickstart their day. You can customize this bowl with their favorite toppings like coconut flakes, chia seeds, and almond butter for added flavor and texture.

For lunch, consider a colorful veggie wrap filled with a variety of fresh vegetables, hummus, and avocado. This meal is not only visually appealing but also packed with vitamins, minerals, and fiber to keep your child feeling full and satisfied. You can also add some grilled chicken or tofu for an extra protein boost.

Dinner time can be a great opportunity to introduce new flavors and ingredients to your child's palate. Try making a homemade vegetable stir-fry with quinoa or brown rice for a nutritious and delicious meal. You can also incorporate superfoods like kale, spinach, and broccoli to provide an extra dose of vitamins and antioxidants.

Snack time is another important aspect of fueling growing minds. Instead of reaching for processed snacks, opt for homemade options like energy balls made with dates, nuts, and seeds. These snacks are not only easy to make but also packed with nutrients to keep your child energized throughout the day.

Remember, the key to fueling growing minds is to provide a variety of nutrient-dense foods that will support your child's overall health and well-being. By incorporating these meal ideas into your child's diet, you can help them reach their full potential and thrive both physically and mentally.

Chapter 9: Sugar-Free Nutrition Food for Kids

Hidden Sugars in Children's Foods

Hidden sugars in children's foods can be a major concern for parents who are trying to provide their little ones with healthy and nutritious meals. While some sugars are naturally occurring in fruits and dairy products, many processed foods aimed at children are loaded with added sugars that can have negative effects on their health. It's important to be aware of these hidden sugars and make informed choices when it comes to feeding your kids.

One of the main culprits when it comes to hidden sugars in children's foods is sugary drinks. Fruit juices, flavored milk, and sports drinks may seem like healthy options, but they often contain high levels of added sugars that can contribute to weight gain and tooth decay. Instead, opt for water or unsweetened beverages to quench your child's thirst without the added sugar.

Another source of hidden sugars in children's foods is breakfast cereals. Many popular brands of cereal marketed towards kids are packed with sugar, even those that claim to be "healthy" or "whole grain." To avoid starting your child's day off with a sugar rush, look for cereals with minimal added sugars or consider making your own homemade granola using natural sweeteners like honey or maple syrup.

Snack foods are another common culprit when it comes to hidden sugars in children's diets. Packaged snacks like granola bars, fruit snacks, and yogurt tubes often contain added sugars to enhance flavor and increase shelf life. Instead, try offering your kids whole foods snacks like fresh fruit, veggies with hummus, or homemade trail mix to satisfy their hunger without the added sugar.

By being mindful of hidden sugars in children's foods and making conscious choices to limit their intake, you can help set your kids up for a lifetime of healthy eating habits. Encourage them to enjoy a variety of nutrient-dense foods that nourish their bodies and support their growth and development. With a little planning and creativity, you can provide your children with delicious and nutritious meals that keep them feeling their best.

Sugar-Free Dessert Options for Kids

Are you looking for healthy and delicious dessert options for your kids that are free from added sugars? Look no further! In this subchapter, we will explore some creative and tasty sugar-free dessert ideas that your kids will love. These desserts are not only good for your child's health but also satisfy their sweet tooth in a nutritious way.

One great sugar-free dessert option for kids is homemade fruit popsicles. Simply blend your child's favorite fruits such as berries, bananas, and mangoes, and pour the mixture into popsicle molds. Freeze them for a few hours and voila! Your kids will have a refreshing and naturally sweet treat that is free from added sugars and artificial ingredients.

Another delicious sugar-free dessert idea for kids is chia seed pudding. Chia seeds are packed with nutrients and when mixed with almond milk, vanilla extract, and a touch of stevia or honey, they create a creamy and satisfying pudding that your kids will love. Top it with fresh berries or nuts for added flavor and texture.

For a fun and healthy twist on traditional dessert, try making banana "nice cream" with your kids. Simply blend frozen bananas with a splash of almond milk and a touch of cocoa powder or vanilla extract. This creamy and indulgent treat tastes just like ice cream but without the added sugars and preservatives.

If your kids love cookies, consider making sugar-free oatmeal cookies using mashed bananas, oats, and a sprinkle of cinnamon. These cookies are a great snack or dessert option for kids and can be easily customized with additions like raisins, nuts, or chocolate chips.

Lastly, consider making sugar-free energy balls with your kids using ingredients like dates, nuts, and coconut flakes. These bite-sized treats are perfect for on-the-go snacking and are a great way to satisfy your child's sweet cravings without any added sugars. Get creative with flavors by adding ingredients like cocoa powder, peanut butter, or dried fruits.

Overall, there are plenty of delicious and nutritious sugar-free dessert options for kids that you can easily make at home. By incorporating these treats into your child's diet, you can promote a healthy relationship with food and teach them the importance of making nutritious choices. So go ahead and get creative in the kitchen with your little ones and enjoy these guilt-free desserts together!

Tips for Reducing Sugar in Kids' Diets

In today's world, it can be challenging to navigate the sea of sugary temptations that surround our children. From sugary cereals to sweet treats, it seems like sugar is everywhere. However, as parents, we have the power to make a positive impact on our kids' health by reducing their sugar intake. Here are some tips for reducing sugar in your kids' diets that will benefit their overall well-being.

First and foremost, it's important to read labels and be mindful of hidden sugars in packaged foods. Many seemingly healthy snacks and drinks contain high amounts of added sugars, which can contribute to weight gain and other health issues. By taking the time to read labels and choose products with lower sugar content, you can help your kids make healthier choices.

Another tip for reducing sugar in your kids' diets is to limit sugary beverages. Sodas, fruit juices, and sports drinks are often loaded with sugar, which can lead to cavities and weight gain. Encourage your kids to drink water or unsweetened beverages instead, and reserve sugary drinks for special occasions.

Additionally, incorporating more whole foods into your kids' diets can help reduce their sugar intake. Fruits, vegetables, whole grains, and lean proteins are all nutritious options that can satisfy their cravings without the added sugars found in processed foods. By focusing on whole foods, you can help your kids develop healthy eating habits that will last a lifetime.

It's also important to lead by example and model healthy eating habits for your kids. If they see you reaching for sugary snacks and drinks, they are more likely to do the same. By making conscious choices to reduce your own sugar intake and opt for nutritious foods, you can set a positive example for your children to follow.

Lastly, getting creative in the kitchen can be a fun way to reduce sugar in your kids' diets. Try experimenting with new recipes and incorporating natural sweeteners like honey, maple syrup, or stevia in place of refined sugars. By making homemade snacks and meals, you can control the ingredients and reduce the amount of sugar your kids consume. Remember, small changes can make a big difference in your kids' health and well-being.

Chapter 10: Probiotic-Rich Nutrition Food for Kids

Benefits of Probiotics for Children's Digestive Health

Probiotics are beneficial bacteria that can have a positive impact on children's digestive health. These friendly bacteria help to maintain a healthy balance in the gut and support the optimal functioning of the digestive system. By including probiotic-rich foods in your child's diet, you can help to promote good gut health and improve overall digestion.

One of the key benefits of probiotics for children is their ability to aid in the digestion and absorption of nutrients. By maintaining a healthy balance of bacteria in the gut, probiotics can help to ensure that your child is able to get the most out of their food and receive all the essential nutrients they need to grow and thrive. This can be particularly important for picky eaters or children with digestive issues who may have trouble absorbing certain nutrients.

In addition to supporting digestion, probiotics can also help to boost the immune system. The gut is home to a large portion of the body's immune cells, and a healthy balance of bacteria is essential for optimal immune function. By including probiotic-rich foods in your child's diet, you can help to strengthen their immune system and reduce their risk of developing infections and illnesses.

Furthermore, probiotics have been shown to have a positive impact on mood and behavior. The gut-brain connection is a powerful one, and research has shown that the health of the gut can have a significant impact on mental health and wellbeing. By supporting good gut health with probiotics, you can help to promote a positive mood and reduce symptoms of anxiety and depression in children.

Overall, incorporating probiotic-rich foods into your child's diet can have a wide range of benefits for their digestive health, immune system, and overall wellbeing. Whether you choose to include probiotics in the form of yogurt, kefir, sauerkraut, or other fermented foods, you can help to support your child's health and vitality with these beneficial bacteria. So why not start adding some probiotic-rich foods to your child's diet today and reap the rewards of improved digestive health and overall wellbeing!

Probiotic-Rich Foods Kids Will Love

Are you looking for ways to incorporate more probiotic-rich foods into your child's diet? Look no further! Probiotics are beneficial bacteria that can help support your child's digestive health and overall well-being. Luckily, there are plenty of delicious options that kids will love.

One popular probiotic-rich food that kids tend to enjoy is yogurt. Yogurt is not only rich in probiotics, but it is also a good source of calcium and protein. You can easily incorporate yogurt into your child's diet by serving it as a snack, adding it to smoothies, or using it as a topping for granola or fruit.

Another kid-friendly probiotic option is kefir. Kefir is a fermented milk drink that is like yogurt but has a thinner consistency. Kids may enjoy the slightly tangy taste of kefir, especially when blended into a tasty smoothie or used as a base for homemade popsicles.

Fermented vegetables, such as sauerkraut and pickles, are also great probiotic-rich foods that kids can enjoy. These foods may have a stronger taste than yogurt or kefir, so it's a good idea to start with small amounts and gradually increase the serving size. You can serve fermented vegetables as a side dish or add them to sandwiches or salads for an extra boost of probiotics.

If your child has a sweet tooth, consider offering them some kombucha. Kombucha is a fizzy, fermented tea that comes in a variety of flavors. Kids may enjoy the bubbly texture and fruity taste of kombucha, making it a fun and tasty way to get their dose of probiotics.

By incorporating these probiotic-rich foods into your child's diet, you can help support their digestive health and overall well-being. Encourage your child to try new foods and flavors, and make mealtimes a fun and exciting experience. With a little creativity and experimentation, you can find delicious ways to boost your child's gut health with probiotic-rich foods they will love.

Incorporating Probiotics into Kids' Daily Routine

Incorporating probiotics into your kids' daily routine is a great way to support their overall health and well-being. Probiotics are beneficial bacteria that help to maintain a healthy balance in the gut, which is essential for a strong immune system and proper digestion. By adding probiotic-rich foods to your child's diet, you can help to promote good gut health and support their overall wellness.

One easy way to incorporate probiotics into your kids' daily routine is by including yogurt in their meals and snacks. Yogurt is a great source of probiotics, and it can be enjoyed on its own or mixed with fruits and nuts for a tasty and nutritious treat. You can also try adding yogurt to smoothies or using it as a base for homemade popsicles for a fun and healthy snack option.

Another way to introduce probiotics to your kids is by incorporating fermented foods into their diet. Foods like sauerkraut, kimchi, and kombucha are all rich in probiotics and can be easily added to meals or enjoyed as a side dish. These foods not only provide a good source of probiotics but also offer a variety of flavors and textures that can help to expand your child's palate.

If your child is not a fan of yogurt or fermented foods, you can also consider giving them a probiotic supplement. There are many options available on the market, including chewable tablets, gummies, and powders that can be easily mixed into water or juice. Just be sure to choose a high-quality supplement that is specifically designed for children and consult with your pediatrician before adding it to their routine.

Overall, incorporating probiotics into your kids' daily routine is a simple and effective way to support their gut health and overall well-being. By making small changes to their diet and lifestyle, you can help to ensure that they are getting the essential nutrients they need to thrive. So why not give probiotics a try and see the positive impact they can have on your child's health and happiness!

Chapter 11: Homemade Nutrition Food for Kids

Advantages of Homemade Meals for Children

Homemade meals for children offer a plethora of advantages that are beneficial for their overall health and well-being. One of the key benefits of preparing meals at home is that it allows you to have complete control over the ingredients that go into your child's food. This means you can ensure that your child is getting all the essential nutrients they need for proper growth and development. By using fresh, organic ingredients, you can provide your child with a nutritionally balanced meal that is free from harmful additives and preservatives.

In addition to being more nutritious, homemade meals are also a great way to introduce children to a variety of flavors and textures. When you cook at home, you have the freedom to experiment with different ingredients and recipes, helping your child develop a diverse palate and a love for healthy foods. By involving your child in the cooking process, you can also teach them valuable skills that will benefit them for a lifetime.

Another advantage of homemade meals for children is that they can be tailored to meet your child's specific dietary needs. Whether your child has food allergies, sensitivities, or specific dietary preferences, cooking at home allows you to accommodate these needs without sacrificing taste or nutrition. You can easily customize recipes to be gluten-free, vegan, sugar-free, or allergy-friendly, ensuring that your child is getting the nourishment they need without any unnecessary restrictions.

Furthermore, homemade meals can help foster a sense of togetherness and connection within your family. Sitting down to a home-cooked meal not only provides an opportunity for bonding and conversation, but it also promotes healthy eating habits and mindfulness around food. By making mealtimes a priority and involving your child in the process, you can instill a lifelong appreciation for good nutrition and the joy of cooking.

Overall, the advantages of homemade meals for children are numerous and undeniable. From providing essential nutrients and fostering a diverse palate to accommodating specific dietary needs and promoting family bonding, cooking at home is a simple yet powerful way to support your child's health and well-being. So why not roll up your sleeves, get cooking, and enjoy the countless benefits of homemade meals with your little ones today!

Easy Recipes for Homemade Baby Food

Are you looking for easy and nutritious recipes to make homemade baby food for your little one? Look no further! In this subchapter, we will provide you with some simple and delicious recipes that are perfect for your baby's developing taste buds. Making your own baby food at home is not only cost-effective but also allows you to control the ingredients and ensure that your little one is getting the best possible nutrition.

First up, we have a simple recipe for homemade apple sauce. All you need to do is peel and core a few apples, chop them into small pieces, and cook them in a saucepan with a little water until they are soft. Then, simply blend the apples until you reach your desired consistency. This apple sauce is not only delicious but also packed with vitamins and fiber that are essential for your baby's growth and development.

Next, we have a recipe for sweet potato puree. Sweet potatoes are a great source of beta-carotene, which is important for your baby's immune system. Simply peel and chop a sweet potato, steam or boil it until it is soft, and then blend it until smooth. You can also add a dash of cinnamon or nutmeg for extra flavor. Your baby will love the natural sweetness of this puree!

For a protein-packed option, try making homemade lentil puree. Lentils are a great source of protein and iron, which are important nutrients for your baby's growth. Simply cook some lentils until they are soft, then blend them with a little water or breast milk until you reach your desired consistency. You can also add some chopped vegetables for added nutrients. Your baby will love the creamy texture of this puree!

If you're looking for a refreshing and nutritious snack for your baby, try making homemade fruit popsicles. Simply blend your favorite fruits, such as strawberries, bananas, and blueberries, with a little water or fruit juice, and pour the mixture into popsicle molds. Freeze them for a few hours until they are solid, and voila! Your baby will love the cool and fruity treat, and you can rest easy knowing that they are getting a healthy snack.

In conclusion, making homemade baby food doesn't have to be complicated or time-consuming. With a few simple ingredients and some creativity, you can provide your little one with delicious and nutritious meals that will support their growth and development. Give these easy recipes a try and watch your baby enjoy every bite!

Cooking with Kids: Fun and Nutritious Recipes to Make Together

Cooking with kids can be a fun and rewarding experience for both parents and children. Not only does it provide an opportunity for quality bonding time, but it also teaches important life skills and encourages a love for healthy eating. In this subchapter, we will explore some fun and nutritious recipes that you can make together with your little ones.

One of the best ways to get kids excited about cooking is to involve them in the process from start to finish. Let them help pick out the ingredients at the store, measure out the portions, and mix everything together. This hands-on approach not only makes cooking more enjoyable for kids, but it also helps them develop a sense of independence and confidence in the kitchen.

When it comes to choosing recipes to make with kids, opt for dishes that are not only delicious but also nutritious. Consider recipes that incorporate a variety of fruits, vegetables, whole grains, and lean proteins. This way, you can ensure that your little ones are getting the essential nutrients they need to grow and thrive.

Some fun and nutritious recipes to try with your kids include homemade veggie pizza, fruit kabobs with yogurt dip, and smoothie bowls topped with nuts and seeds. These dishes are not only easy to make, but they also provide a good balance of carbohydrates, protein, and healthy fats. Plus, they are sure to be a hit with even the pickiest eaters!

Remember, cooking with kids is not just about making meals – it's about creating memories and instilling healthy habits that will last a lifetime. So put on your aprons, roll up your sleeves, and get ready to have some fun in the kitchen with your little ones!

Conclusion: Empowering Parents to Nourish Their Kids with Healthy Foods

In conclusion, empowering parents to nourish their kids with healthy foods is essential for their overall well-being and development. As parents, you have the power to shape your child's eating habits and set them up for a lifetime of good health. By providing nutritious and balanced meals, you are giving your child the fuel they need to thrive physically, mentally, and emotionally.

It is important to remember that every bite counts when it comes to your child's nutrition. By incorporating a variety of foods from different food groups, you can ensure that your child is getting all the essential nutrients they need to grow and thrive. From fruits and vegetables to whole grains and lean proteins, each food group plays a vital role in your child's health.

As you navigate the world of nutrition food for kids, whether it be organic, vegan, gluten-free, or allergy-friendly options, remember that there is no one-size-fits-all approach. It's about finding what works best for your child and their unique dietary needs. Experiment with new recipes, flavors, and ingredients to keep meals exciting and enjoyable for your little ones.

By focusing on superfood nutrition food for kids, you can provide your child with an extra boost of vitamins, minerals, and antioxidants that can support their immune system and brain health. Don't forget the importance of probiotic-rich foods to promote good gut health and sugar-free options to reduce the risk of developing health issues later in life.

In closing, remember that you are not alone in this journey. Seek support from other parents, nutritionists, and healthcare professionals to ensure that you are making the best choices for your child's nutrition. By empowering yourself with knowledge and taking small steps each day, you can set your child up for a lifetime of good health and happiness.

9 798329 864977